ARE YOU DOING IT THE RIGHT WAY?

Let's Kickstart Fitness – Beginners Guide

MORTUZA KARZON

Contents

INTRODUCTION

At the mention of the word "fitness", what comes to your mind? Whatever you think concerning the word will be different from anybody's thought. You can do a simple experiment by asking 10 individuals what fitness means to them. Their response will be totally different. For some, it entails going to the gym lifting weights or making use of cardio machines. For others, it may mean participating in an aerobics class. If you are among those with this thought, it is time to think twice because I can guarantee you that you have things mixed up.

We hear the word "fitness" daily so much that we mix up what it really means. Have you ever taken the time to think what does fitness mean? Fitness is more about enjoying your life. It has numerous benefits associated with it, which is why everyone is concerned about it. Ask an overweight individual who is now in shape the importance of fitness and you won't be surprised by their response. Fitness helps you in burning calories, relieving stress, improving disposition, getting better sleep, less sickness, and much more. In this eBook on bodybuilding for beginners, you will learn the basic strength training, strategies for strength training, bodybuilding techniques for beginners, powerlifting techniques, 12-weeks bodybuilding plan and much more.

In antediluvian times, we had no elliptical machines, motorized treadmills, or exercise bikes. There was nothing like weight machines or free weights. Nevertheless, this doesn't mean that people weren't fit. Of course, they kept fit because fitness is a way of living. Farming, foraging, and maintaining a home requires people to move constantly. They may not have any form of structured workout routines; it didn't mean they suffered from health problems common today. They ate every natural food from the ground and sustained a daily high-calorie burnout. Combining these two factors gives them a healthy body and made they fit – strong, agile, and lean.

Consider every sort of natural fitness you have been doing right from childhood. An active, healthy child usually doesn't spend time at the gym lifting weights or on the treadmills. Rather, children play and run around but enjoy it. The same applies with every fitness regime you try to integrate into your daily activity.

WHERE WE ARE TODAY

So, what is the definition of fitness? For most people, it encompasses going to the gym. Nowadays, we work in an office where we remain inactive for hours and in the evening after a little activity, we get to bed. Our routine becomes the consumption of high-calorie processed foods with inactive activities. Can this be connected to the numerous health challenges we face in life?

No matter how you may see it, it is connected. Fitness is important to your overall health and reaping these benefits comes with a mindset change of what fitness entails. What are the key advantages of sticking to a regular fitness program?

HEALTH BENEFIT OF FITNESS

- Lower blood pressure

- Reduced risk of sickness

- Increased bone density

- Increased muscle strength

- Lower resting heart rate

- Reduced risk of injuries

- Improved insulin sensitivity

- Enhanced glucose tolerance

- Lower body fat level and body weight

- Improved cardiovascular function

- Reduced stress level

- Reduced risk of mass loss

- Improved posture

- Improved sleep quality

- Reduced anxiety

- Reduced risk of developing depression

- Improved body image and self-confidence

- Stronger muscles

- Reduced appearance of body fat

With this, you have a brief introduction of what fitness is and the benefits associated with it. Fitness encompasses three basic elements

- Strength Training

- Flexibility training

- Cardiovascular training

In the next chapter, we will unravel the strength training for beginners. Strength can be actualized via the traditional weightlifting programs or any bodybuilding activity. With this basic introduction, it is believed that you have the foundational knowledge of fitness. It is time to learn something more fun!

KEYS TO ACCOMPLISHING FITNESS

As a beginner to fitness, there are important basic things that will fast track your goal and put you in shape for your various fitness training. They are like the alphabets, which you must know, else you cannot understand how words are formed.

No Particular type of training: Only when you are training for marathon else you don't have to spend countless hours repeating the same exercise. Integrate other training into it. Training such as stretching, plyometric, swimming, sprinting, bodyweight/calisthenics (dips, pull-ups, push-ups, etc.), yoga, cycling, jogging, lifting, and more. Just mix them up.

No "schedules": Don't form the habit of creating a routine when it comes to fitness. You don't have to jog every Tuesday or every day. Spice up your fitness training with something new constantly as you learn in what way, your body reacts. This will make it easier for you.

Cross-Train: There is no need training every day. Play different kind of sports such as football, soccer, hockey, basketball. You can also go out with your kids or nephews and have fun.

Set goals: To help you stay on track, you must set goals. Goals are important not just for your fitness purpose but in life in general. You can set short, medium and long-term goals. Perhaps your goal may be working out every three hours for a week, work towards it and you will make it.

Keep records of your progress: After setting a goal, you need to keep track of it. You can use your computer or notebook. Nowadays, we have apps for phones that enable you to keep your workout records. As time goes on, measure your accomplishment with the goal set.

CHAPTER ONE: STRENGTH 101

Yes, you have read the various benefits of fitness to your overall health but it won't do you any good without putting action to it. You must be committed to a particular fitness program. This will help in making positive changes in your body. As with most beginners, they are always puzzled by the question, where do I start? Well, the first place to begin is "strength training." It is the foundation of fitness. Strength training has great benefits, especially when followed practically. Within a short a time, you could see the drastic transformation in your body.

Though strength training is the foundation of fitness, yet people tend to shy away from it because of two major reasons. Firstly, is their uncertainty in how strength training is performed correctly and secondly, the fear of developing bulky muscles. For most men, having a bulky muscle is great. Some women would rather prefer maintaining their feminine image and because of this, avoid strength training. If you still hold this perspective as a woman, it is time to do away with it because strength training is an integral aspect of exercising for a woman. Strength training will not make you have bulky muscles because as a woman you don't have the amount of testosterone to do so. Therefore, strength training is for everyone both male and female.

Studies have shown that strength training can make you feel and look better. It also helps you in losing weight. Strength training isn't about bodybuilders going to the gym to lift weights. It is beneficial to all group of people – old and young. If you know anyone suffering from health issues like heart condition or arthritis, strength training is helpful. The following are some of the benefits of strength training.

Protects your muscle mass and bone health

After adolescence, whether you are a woman or man, you start losing a percent of your muscle strength and bone per year. The best way of preventing, stopping or reversing your muscle loss is by integrating a strength training into your workout routine.

Makes you fitter and stronger

Strength training involves the toning and strengthening of your muscles through the contraction of the muscles by a resisting force. This is why strength training is also called "resistance training

Help you develop a better body mechanics

The benefits of strength training go beyond the physical. It helps in improving the coordination and balance of your body including your posture. For those with poor body balance and flexibility, strength training help in reducing your risk of falling by 40 percent. This is an important benefit for anyone even as people get old.

Strength Training helps in prevention of disease

People suffering from arthritis can use strength training to reduce the pain. Strength training is an effective medication that has used in reducing arthritis pain. Also, for post-menopausal women, strength training help in reducing the risk of bone fractures while increasing their bone density. A healthy lifestyle with strength training will help in improving the glucose control for people suffering from type 2 diabetes.

Improves and boost your mode and energy level respectively

Strength training helps in increasing the level of endorphins in your brain, making you feel better. Studies have also shown that it is a good antidepressant for those looking for a good sleep. if you want to improve the quality of your life, consider mixing strength training into your workout routine.

STRENGTH TRAINING: GETTING STARTED

One of the mistakes beginners does is limiting themselves to the gym, expensive machines or lifting weights as the primary ways of doing strength training. Lunges, jump squats, pushups, and mountain climbing are examples of strength training.

Note: Before getting involved in any kind of strength training, ensure there are no health issues with you. Consult your doctor to certify you can undergo any fitness exercise.

TYPES OF STRENGTH TRAINING

Strength training comes in many types and determining the particular one to integrate into your workout routine may be a challenge. Is there a widely accepted way to strength training? Which strength training is best suited for you? Does one method have an advantage over the other?

Some of these questions will be answered in this section. However, the first thing is defining your workout goals. It is not enough saying you want to lose weight; you must be specific. It has to be something quantifiable. You must set a goal like "losing 10 pounds on your next anniversary." The following are the important 5 types of strength training you should know about.

Total Body Circuit Training

This strength training is a traditional boot camp-style workout program like the Insanity and P90x programs. Using this type of strength training involves you using a lightweight in different motion to work out every aspect of your body.

Who can do this training? As a beginner, this training is good for you because it ensures you don't feel much pain in your muscle. It is the best method of achieving a moderate weight within a certain period.

Push-Pull Training

From the name, it is a description of how it works. For a start, you can break down the body into three basic movement plains: the muscles that pull, the muscles that push and everything in your lower body. Dividing your body this way enables certain muscles to rest during the day while you work on others. Each day you allocate a particular work out to each muscle. For instance, your push up days may comprise of shoulders, chest, and triceps. For the pull-up days, you may work on your traps, biceps, and back.

Who can do this training? This particular strength training is essential for those considering developing strength in their entire body. It is perfect for experienced yogis and advanced lifters with good muscles.

Power Lifting Training

This strength training is popular among the ones mentioned here. In gyms today, you will see power racks while some are focused on Cross Fit (powerlifting). In this aspect of strength training, you indulge in larger movements to compliment additional muscles. For instance, exercises such as power cleans, snatches, deadlifts, and squats add more muscle.

Who can do this training? This strength training is not for beginners like you but an advanced method of strength training. When fully incorporated into your workout, the benefits will be evident for all to see. Nevertheless, there is need to be careful when doing this training because of the high risk involved. Looking for a way to build more muscle while reducing fat at no cost, then you must integrate powerlifting training into your workout routine.

Explosive Dynamic Training

Most athletes do this type of strength training. An example includes rope pulls, box jumps, and lighter weight powerlifting movements like cleans, snatches, and squats. As a beginner, you may think there is no difference between this training and powerlifting; however, the key difference lies in the rate at which you work out fast. This enables you to do your strength and cardio workout concurrently.

Who can do this training? This is your perfect program for dropping some pounds of weight quickly instead of using drugs. Training at a higher rate leads to your heart rate beating high, which will remove unwanted weight. You will also experience changes in your muscle and burn off more calories.

Muscular Isolation Training

In this strength training, for a particular day, you work with only one or two muscle groups. The aim of this training is to cause muscular contraction of a particular muscle. Exercises such as triceps kickbacks, concentration curls, and leg extension are what you will do in this training.

Who can do this training? It is good for beginners and advanced lifters in developing particular muscle groups

No matter what your goal may be, there is a perfect strength training to suit your needs.

PRINCIPLES TO START STRENGTH TRAINING

Start small

Most beginners make this mistake by starting big. Your loved ones need your attention. Because your attention is divided, for some time you haven't gone to the gym. Start small! 20 minutes a day is a good way to start. As you keep to it, it becomes a habit and before you know, you hit the gym always. Don't rush it. Take it slow like the snail. Remember you are adding a new habit and habits take time before form. Even if you miss out some days, dust yourself up and continue. The idea is getting the habit of strength training into you.

Be patient

Why do you want to do strength training? What is your aim? Are you doing it because you want to build your body or to intimidate others? Irrespective what your aim may be, patience is required. We live in a world where everything is instantaneous, so I won't blame you if you want to rush your strength training. Anyone that tells you that strength training is a skill that can be mastered a day or week is merely deceiving you. Strength training requires consistent practice. It is just like footballers; they need to practice constantly. Approach strength training like an artist takes his time to paint his greatest masterpiece. The Little step of improvement will overhaul your body to how you want it.

Begin with bodyweight movements

Have you ever seen someone who buys a house with a weak foundation? Will you want to go to a surgeon who never went to medical school? Every foundation is very important – no matter how small or big it may be. Your body isn't different with strength training. If you are looking for a superstructure, build the foundation sturdy. Practice bodyweight movements.

Choose compound movements instead of isolation movements

Most people don't have time to "waste" in the gym which is why the particular exercise selected must be precise. Compound exercises include chin-ups, deadlifts, squats, and hip thrust enables the muscle groups to work concurrently while burning out calories unlike the isolation exercises like bicep curls, kickbacks, triceps, and the hip abductor machine.

Concentrate on getting stronger

Whether you are a girl or guy who wants extra lean muscle, your main priority should be increasing your strength working out goal. You are not going to build your body by lifting light reps but challenging weights will build your body quickly. This will provide you a firm foundation for your workout activity. Though it may be frightening for most women to lift challenging weights, however, women don't carry adequate hormonal testosterone to build muscles as their male counterparts do. Aside from pain management, improved stability, and bone health, lifting weights is a way of relieving stress.

Think quality over quantity

When doing your strength training, it is not about the quantity of training done but the quality. Select quality exercises rather than selecting a variety of exercises just to keep yourself busy. A compound lift of 30 minutes is of more quality than a 90-minute workout that comprises of long rest periods and isolation exercises. Your motor should be Get in Getting Out!

Prioritize form

You may not have heard this but you should prioritize your form above everything. Whatever workout routine you are performing, ensure that particular muscle is working. Drop your ego and pride at your doorstep and focus on the technique to get the best results possible. Prioritize your form.

STRATEGIES FOR STRENGTH TRAINING

There have been different strength training techniques over the years with most of them faded away. Finding the right strategy to strength training isn't easy; however, this eBook has everything you need regarding the right strategy for strength training as a beginner. In this section, we will discuss important training strategies to gain the optimal amount of muscle you can within the shortest time possible. These strategies have been around but never followed in their right way. Let us look at them.

Training Frequency

The intensity of your strength training exercise and the recovery after the exercise are two important component of strength training. To increase your functional muscle size within the shortest time requires a short, infrequent, and high-intensity weight training sessions trailed with the needed recovery time. Your strength training is not about the volume but the recuperation and intensity when it comes to gaining muscle and strength.

Exercises for each Session

According to studies, you have a limited amount of energy needed during a weight training session. Various tests were used during this study including the blood test of individuals. The blood test also revealed a dropping of the blood sugar level after 20 to 30 minutes of high-intensity training. Since you have a little time to train before your blood sugar level drops, this makes the choice of exercise crucial. You can use compound or multi-joint movements because you can train different muscles concurrently.

Number of Repetitions per Set

The growth of strength and muscle is interconnected. Strength training sessions result to increase in strength, which is equivalent to increase in functional muscle. What this means is that you will grow muscle and become stronger.

STRENGTH TRAINING TIPS FOR BEGINNERS

For a fitness newbie, strength training can be intimidating especially if you have never worked on the levers and pulleys. Nevertheless, a crucial aspect of being fit is strength training and you cannot ignore this. You have read about the benefits of strength training and knowing these 5 tips as a beginner will help you towards your fitness goal.

Do cardio Warm-up

Prior to your starting your strength training, warming your heart beat rate is very important. You can start with 5 minutes dynamic stretching, light jogging or brisk walking. Dynamic stretching involves organized movements aim to increase your range of motion and loosen your muscles. Ensure you do some butt kicks and walking lunges.

Learn proper technique

To avoid any form of injuries, ensure you know the right technique and form to use. Using the right technique will ascertain that the right muscles are working and not strained. If you are actually a beginner, investing in a single training session will be beneficial to you. A trainer can help you by showing you the right motions, grips, and positions. If you don't want to invest money by hiring a trainer, you may find online content that offers free training.

Know your options

There are many options available to you like using dumbbells with your strength training. Actually, in the gym, there are modes of strength training you can do. You can use weight bars, exercise balls, medicine balls, kettlebells, resistance bands or your own body weight. You can learn a lot in strength training classes because these classes offer you the best way of learning how to use the equipment in the gym.

Know the right weight for yourself

As a beginner, this may be hard for you but with constant experimentation, you can know the accurate weight suitable for you. It is better as a beginner to err on little weight than too heavyweight. For instance, if you are doing 4 sets of 12 reps of bicep curls, during the last set, your arms will feel fatigued.

Allow your routine to evolve

Once you become familiar with strength training, it is imperative to integrate equipment and new exercises into your workout routine. Spice up each session and ensure you monitor the amount of weight you raise.

CHAPTER TWO: BODYBUILDING TECHNIQUES FOR BEGINNERS

ELEMENT OF BODYBUILDING

There is nothing like a perfect bodybuilding weight training routine for all size, but with certain principles, you can maximize the result. In this section, you will learn how to incorporate periodization, progressive overload, and exercise variety into your weight training routine. Symmetry and proportion are an important element of bodybuilding. The "total package" you want is achievable by combining the key element.

Periodization

This is the idea of changing exercise variables such as frequency, intensity, and volume over time to maximize your training progress. This enables you to train at a high volume or intensity with changing periods of lower volume or intensity to improve your recovery time while maximizing your performance. There are different periodization models to use but the common one is the linear periodization. This involves decreasing the reps/volume while increasing the intensity/weight every 4-6weeks. For instance, in phase one you have 15 reps with 100lbs, in phase two, it will be 12 reps with 110lbs, followed by phase three with 10 reps of 120lbs and finally phase four with 8 reps with 130lbs.

Progressive Overload

You will not experience any improvement if you use the same amount of resistance for the same number of reps in your workout. Progressive overload involves the gradual increase of the body's demand during exercise to increase the muscle mass and strength. Try increasing resistance, reps, sets, training frequency, or the number of exercises you do every 6-8 weeks to ensure muscular overload in your training program.

12-WEEK BODYBUILDING PLAN FOR BEGINNERS

To help you actualize this 12-week bodybuilding plan as a beginner, we have divided it into four different phases, which is split into three weeks. Without further ado, let us begin!

PHASE 1 (WEEK 1-3)

You don't need the IQ of Einstein to guess that doing a general body training requires training your entire body. This is ideal for beginners because it enables them to train each muscle group each week. You can do this training three times a week – Monday, Wednesday, and Friday. The benefit of this repetition training is to help train the body's nervous system.

It is advisable to do this training thrice a week to enable you to rest a day between each training. Your body needs to recoup after the previous workout. To become stronger and bigger, the recovery process is important.

Workouts	Sets	Rest Time
Barbell Bench Press	3 sets of 10-12 reps	2-3 minutes rest
Bent-Over Barbell Row	3 Sets of 10-12 reps	2-3 minutes rest
Squat	3 Sets of 10-12 reps	2-3 minutes rest
Barbell Shoulder Press	3 Sets of 10-12 reps	2-3 minutes rest
Triceps Push-Down	3 Sets of 10-12 reps	2-3 minutes rest
Barbell Curl	3 Sets of 10-12 reps	2-3 minutes rest
Standing Calf Raise	3 Sets of 10-12 reps	2-3 minutes rest
Crunch	3 Sets of 10-12 reps	2-3 minutes rest

Phase 1 Explanation

EXERCISES

You will be using the tried-and-true mass builders' exercises, which include barbell curl, squat, bench press, etc. You will be doing one exercise for each muscle group for this phase.

REPS

This is an acronym for repetition and it involves performing a particular exercise once through its full range of motion. During this phase, as a beginner, you should aim for 10-12 reps per set. For beginners, this is the good range to build the strength and size of a body.

WEIGHT

Your rep range determines the amount of weight you use. Since you will be doing about 10-12 reps for each set, it is better to choose a weight that enables you to do not less than 10 reps or more than 12 reps. You should grow stronger over these three weeks.

SETS

A set means performing all the reps for an exercise. This involves picking up the bar and doing as many reps possible before you drop the bar completes one set. Normally, several sets per exercise can be done with resting intervals between those sets.

REST

Between each set, there is a resting period of 2-3 minutes. The objective of resting is to enable you to stick fairly close to the rep range through the same weight on all three sets. This is crucial as it supports you to gain more strength and size.

PHASE 2 (WEEK 4-6)

After three weeks of complete body training in the first phase, your muscles are in for a new challenge. For the next three weeks, you will be following a two-day training split twice a week repeatedly. A two-day training divided into two separate workouts. In the first workout, you will train all the torso muscle groups (back, abs, chest, and shoulder) while in the second, you will train all the limb muscles (calves, legs, triceps, and biceps).

Workout 1

Workouts	Sets	Rest Time
Bench Press	3 Sets of 8-10 reps	2-3 minutes rest
Incline Dumbbell Flies	3 Sets of 8-10 reps	2-3 minutes rest

Barbell Row   3 Sets of 8-10 reps   2-3 minutes rest

Lat Pull-down 3 Sets of 10-12 reps   2-3 minutes rest

Barbell shoulder press 3 Sets of 8-10 reps   2-3 minutes rest

Dumbbell Lateral Raise   3 Sets of 10-12 reps   2-3 minutes rest

Barbell Shrug 3 Sets of 8-10 reps   2-3 minutes rest

Reverse Crunch   3 sets to failure   1-2 minutes rest

Crunches   3 sets to failure   1-2 minutes rest

Workout 2

Workout   Sets   Rest Time

Barbell Curl   3 Sets of 8-10 reps   2-3 minutes rest

Incline Dumbbell Curl   3 Sets of 10-12 reps   2-3 minutes rest

Close-Grip Bench Press   3 Sets of 8-10 reps   2-3 minutes rest

Triceps Press down   3 Sets of 10-12 reps   2-3 minutes rest

Squat   3 Sets of 8-10 reps   2-3 minutes rest

Leg Extensions   3 Sets of 10-12 reps   2-3 minutes rest

Lying Leg Curls   3 Sets of 10-12 reps   2-3 minutes rest

Standing Calf Raises 2 Sets of 15-20 reps   2-3 minutes rest

Seated Calf Raise   2 Sets of 15-20 reps   2-3 minutes rest

Phase 2 Explanation

EXERCISES

In this phase, you will focus on the mass builders you begin in the first phase with an additional exercise for that same muscle group. You may be able to work on a new muscle group during this phase especially the trapezium and kite-shaped muscle at the base of your neck.

SETS

You will continue with the three sets per exercise; nevertheless, since for each muscle group you were doing two to three exercises, the total sets will now be from 3 per muscle group to 6 or 9 for legs.

REPS

Your reps will drop to 8-10 during this phase for each muscle group. This will enable you to train heavier than the previous phase. The outcome will be more muscle mass and more strength. You should keep the reps at 1-12 for the second and third exercise.

WEIGHT

During this phase, look for a weight that limits you to 8-10 reps during the first exercise and once that will allow you to make complete 10-12 reps within the second and third exercises.

REST

In this second phase, you need between 2-3 minutes rest between each set. This will enable you to stick with heavier weight and finish more reps for increasing strength and size gain.

PHASE 3 (WEEKS 7-9)

Getting interesting! After following 6 weeks of consistent training, you should congratulate yourself for a job well done. By now, your muscle fibers and nervous system are getting properly trained through the constant repetition. In week nine, you will be stepping up the amount of work for each muscle group. Don't forget the objective is to keep progressing. There is no other way of doing this than raising the bar with high intensity and more work.

Workout 1: Push Day

Workouts	Sets	Rest Time
Bench Press	3 Sets of 6-8 reps	2-3 minutes rest
Incline Dumbbell Press	3 Sets of 8-10 reps	2-3 minutes rest
Incline Dumbbell Flies	3 Sets of 12-15 reps	2-3 minutes rest
Barbell Shoulder Press	3 Sets of 6-8 reps	2-3 minutes rest
Smith Machine Upright Row	3 sets of 8-10 reps	2-3 minutes rest
Dumbbell Lateral Raise	3 Sets of 12-15 reps	2-3 minutes rest

Close-Grip Bench Press   3 Sets of 6-8 reps   2-3 minutes rest

Dumbbell Overhead Triceps Extension   3 Sets of 8-10 reps   2-3 minutes rest

Triceps Press down   3 Sets of 12-15 reps   2-3 minutes rest

Workout 2: Legs Day

Squat   3 Sets of 6-8 reps   2-3 minutes rest

Leg Press   3 Sets of 8-10 reps   2-3 minutes rest

Leg Extensions   3 Sets of 12-15 reps   2-3 minutes rest

Lying Leg Curls   3 Sets of 12-15 reps   2-3 minutes rest

Standing Calf Raises 3 Sets of 20-25 reps   1-2 minutes rest

Seated Calf Raise   3 Sets of 20-25 reps   1-2 minutes rest

Reverse Crunch   3 Sets to failure   1-2 minutes rest

Crunches   3 Sets to failure   1-2 minutes rest

Oblique Crunches   3 Sets to Failure   1-2 minutes rest

Workout 3: Pull Day

Barbell Row   3 Sets of 6-8 reps   2-3 minutes rest

Lat Pulldown 3 Sets of 8-10 reps   2-3 minutes rest

Seated Cable Rows   3 Sets of 12-15 reps   2-3 minutes rest

Barbell Shrug 3 Sets of 6-8 reps   2-3 minutes rest

Barbell Curl   3 Sets of 6-8 reps   2-3 minutes rest

Incline Dumbbell Curl   3 Sets of 8-10 reps   2-3 minutes rest

Preacher Curl 3 Sets of 12-15 reps   2-3 minutes rest

Wrist Curl   3 Sets of 10-12 reps   1-2 minutes rest

Phase 3 Explanation

EXERCISES

This exercise in this phase isn't different from those of the previous phases; however, you will add another exercise to most of the muscle groups. The idea is to increase the workload for each muscle group.

SETS

You will be performing 3 sets for each exercise. Nevertheless, you will be doing an additional 3 sets per muscle group since you are adding another exercise for most muscle groups.

REPS

The reps for this phase will drop to 6-8 for the first exercise for each of the key muscle group apart from the forearms, abs, and calves. On the second exercise, the reps should be drop to 8-10. But for the last exercise, consider increasing the reps to 12-15 each set. This will aid the development of the muscle strength, muscle definition, and the muscle size.

WEIGHT

Like in phase 1 and 2, select the proper weight, which will allow you to hit the listed rep range for each exercise.

REST

Like in the previous phases, ensure you rest for 2-3 minutes between each set.

PHASE 4 (WEEK 10-12)

If you made it to this point, congratulation. It means you are on the right track to building your body. It is worth congratulating you after 9 weeks of consistent training involving a gradual progression. You are becoming an advanced bodybuilder; you are just a step away from that. If you were true to yourself, you will experience muscle definition and muscle strength. Don't worry, you are in the final phase of this 12-week bodybuilding plan.

In this final phase, you will be training your entire body with over four-workout course to perform. This will help you in increasing the workload for each muscle group. The training will be split into four days, which will be split into four part of the body – legs and calves' workout; forearms, back, and biceps workout; triceps, chest, and abs workout; and traps, shoulders, and abs workout. Abs workout is done twice for each week because it helps in maintaining your upright posture.

Workout 1

Workout   Sets   Rest Time

Bench Press   3 Sets of 4-6 reps   2-3 minutes rest

Dumbbell Incline Bench   3 Sets of 6-8 reps   2-3 minutes rest

Incline Dumbbell Flies   3 Sets of 15-20 reps   1 minute rest

Cable Crossover   3 Sets of 15-20 reps   1 minute rest

Close-Grip Bench Press   3 Sets of 4-6 reps   2-3 minutes rest

Dumbbell Overhead Triceps Extension   3 Sets of 6-8 reps   2-3 minutes rest

Triceps Press down   3 Sets of 15-20 reps   1 minute rest

Hanging Leg Raise   3 Sets to failure   1 minute rest

Bicycle Crunch   3 Sets to failure   1 minute rest

Plank   3 Sets of 1-minute holds   1 minute rest

Workout 2

Barbell Row   3 Sets of 4-6 reps   2-3 minutes rest

Lat Pulldown 3 Sets of 6-8 reps   2-3 minutes rest

Seated Cable Rows   3 Sets of 15-20 reps   1 minute rest

Barbell Curl   3 Sets of 4-6 reps   2-3 minutes rest

Incline Dumbbell Curl   3 Sets of 6-8 reps   2-3 minutes rest

Preacher Curl 3 Sets of 15-20 reps   1 minute rest

Wrist Curl   3 Sets of 12-15 reps   1 minute rest

Reverse-Grip Wrist Curl   3 Sets of 12-15 reps   1 minute rest

Workout 3

Squat   3 Sets of 4-6 reps   2-3 minutes rest

Leg Press   3 Sets of 4-6 reps   2-3 minutes rest

Leg Extensions   3 Sets of 15-20 reps   1 minute rest

Romanian Deadlift   3 Sets of 4-6 reps   2-3 minutes rest

Lying Leg Curls   3 Sets of 15-20 reps   1 minute rest

Standing Calf Raises 3 Sets of 25-30 reps   1 minute rest

Seated Calf Raise   3 Sets of 25-30 reps   1 minute rest

Workout 4

Barbell Shoulder Press   3 Sets of 4-6 reps   2-3 minutes rest

Smith Machine Upright Row 3 Sets of 6-8 reps   2-3 minutes rest

Dumbbell Lateral Raise   3 Sets of 15-20 reps   1 minute rest

Dumbbell Rear Delt Raise   3 Sets of 15-20 reps   1 minute rest

Barbell Shrug 3 Sets of 4-6 reps   2-3 minutes rest

Reverse Crunch   3 Sets to failure   1 minute rest

Crunches   3 Sets to failure   1 minute rest

Oblique Crunches   3 Sets of 15-20 reps   1 minute rest

Phase 4 Explanation

EXERCISES

This phase comprises of exercises done in previous phases but with additional exercise added. You don't need to add the biceps and triceps exercises.

SETS

Perform 3 sets for each exercise. Nevertheless, you will be adding additional 3 sets because of the additional exercise for most muscle groups.

REPS

In the first exercise, drop the reps to 4-6 per set for each muscle group with exception to the forearms, abs, and calves. This will increase your strength gain. For the second exercise, the rep should be drop to 6-8 reps per set for muscle mass and building strength and muscle mass.

WEIGHT

As performed in the previous 3 phases, ensure you select the right weight for each exercise to enable you to hit the listed rep range.

REST

In this phase like the previous ones, you rest 2-3 minutes between each set when using heavier weight and fewer reps.

CHAPTER THREE: POWERLIFTING TRAINING FOR BEGINNERS

At a point, you may have seen a guy passing through the street or in the gym with beards and loads up a barbell loaded with many 45lb plates. You can see the steel bending literally and this sends shockwaves of awesomeness through the floor with impressive squats you have ever seen. Moreover, you thought within yourself, "how in the hell was that possible?" The answer is powerlifting.

We know you have learned a lot on bodybuilding but it is important to note that the two are not the same. Bodybuilding lay emphases on the pursuit of a particular physique unlike powerlifting, which is a sport of achieving raw strength as humanly possible.

What is the difference between bodybuilding and powerlifting?

Many people tend to believe that bodybuilding and powerlifting are terms interchangeably used. While they both offer a great workout, it is important to note that they are not the same. They are a different bot in their goals and their measurement of success. Undoubtedly, they both use endurance and strength, the effect is different on the body. To help you, we have broken the key difference and some similarities between the two.

Bodybuilding and powerlifting are both intense disciplines with the aim of different measurable outcomes. Bodybuilding is a 24/7 attempt, which requires razor focus. Bodybuilding requires one to utilize cardio, bulking, strength training, and cutting to create the perfect body form.

Unlike powerlifters, bodybuilders make use of exercise to sculpt their body and increase the muscle definition, size, and symmetry. Another key difference between the powerlifting and bodybuilding is that bodybuilding involves the use of 6 to 12 reps with moderate weights. Powerlifting, on the other hand, uses heavier weight and lower reps.

What does it mean to be a powerlifter?

On the outside, powerlifting seems something simple. All you need is to develop as much strength humanly possible using the three fundamental lifts, which are deadlift, bench press, and the low-bar back squat. Towards the end, we will expound on these three in detail. Powerlifters develop a form of mystic sense concerning their training if you stay close to them and as a beginner, you must have this at the back of your mind. Like Ironman triathletes and marathon runners, powerlifters function at the fierce edge of their physical ability.

Powerlifting is extremely taxing and demanding, both mentally and physically. You cannot fake powerlifting. It is just you and your barbell. As a beginner, if your goal is going beyond exercising and dedicating yourself towards the pursuit of hardcore strength, then you can enjoy the rewarding aspect of powerlifting.

You have a lot to learn as a beginner in powerlifting such as bar position, activation, head position, eye gaze, optimal foot position, breathing, rooting, and bracing. Undoubtedly, it is rewarding if you keep to your goal, you will be rewarded.

BENEFITS OF POWERLIFTING TRAINING

Besides gaining muscle strength, there are numerous advantages of powerlifting. When you lift heavy weights, it increases your bone density, which then minimizes the risk of developing osteoporosis and brittle bones in future. It also works for every muscle group within the body doing a compound movement, which improves coordination and develops the large muscle groups. Performing powerlifting training also increases your muscle density, which burns additional fat as you rest and without any effort of losing weight. Powerlifting enables you to get stronger, which reduces the risk of injury and improve your overall wellbeing.

THE FUNDAMENTALS OF POWERLIFTING

When we talk about powerlifting training, our primary focus is on the three basic moves performed in most powerlifting competitions. These moves, which you already know, are the squat, deadlift, and the bench press. We will talk about each to them

You need to perform these three different moves at least once in a week. To begin, you need to test your current level. The general rule is to test your five-rep max in the three lifts and with the number inputted in a rep calculator. This will give you the projected maxes. As a beginner who uses a 5-rep max will experience increase when compared to someone at the intermediate level.

Squat

This involves all the muscles in your body and it brings a sense of achievement when you are able to lift a bar on your back. The squat is a versatile exercise, which you can use for different rep ranges and goals. Squatting enables you to build your muscle and strength while helping you to lose fat. It may be difficult since you are a beginner to determine how to rate it.

How do you rate?

•	Beginner 1 x bodyweight

•	Intermediate 1.5 x Bodyweight

- Advanced 2 x Bodyweight

What is the Perfect Form?

First, you stand up straight holding the bar on your back while your feet are turned out slightly. To start the movement, bend at the knees and hips concurrently. While keeping your weight on your heels with your chest up, lower gradually until your hips stay below your knees. After this, you can push your knees out knees out slightly at the bottom of the squat. This will help you to get additional depth. Then move your knees back in to begin the push back up.

Expert tip

Continue a repeatable process, which will help you go through a mental checklist of cues each time you are ready for a squat. Ensure you grip the bar very tight while pulling the bar down into you. Then stand tall while setting your foot position and posture then begin the squatting. To know if you are doing it according to prescription, you can record yourself and watch it later.

What should I do if I am struggling with performing the squat well?

In the event were getting low becomes an issue, it is advisable to do a pause squats beside a regular mobility routine. Stopping at the bottom will help in slowly releasing the tightness and build strength. It will also give you a good awareness of the exact position.

Bench Press

If you perform the bench press correctly, the effect will be evident in your lats, triceps, delts, and chest. This is the reason why in your powerlifting training, you must add the bench press movement. You can use it to improve your power, strength, build your muscle, and improve your overall fitness. The bench press training is a vital aspect of your upper body exercising.

How do you rate?

Beginner 0.75 x Bodyweight

Intermediate 1 x Bodyweight

Advanced 1.5 x Bodyweight

What is the Perfect form?

According to professionals in powerlifting, the best way of doing the bench press is by "using a bench, lie on your back with your feet stationed on the floor just behind your knees. Then hold the bar with your hands in a way that it is a litter wider than your shoulder width apart. Then lower the bar towards your chest. Press your head and shoulders into the bench and your feet into the floor, and press the bar back up."

Expert tip

Your shoulders blades should be kept in a retracted position while you push through your heels. Using this technique as a beginner will make a lot of difference when doing the bench press training.

Why people get it wrong

One of the mistakes performed by beginners when doing the bench press is the failure in realizing the function of the lower body in the exercise. To correct this, it is important that, "Your legs should provide an additional force to help press the bar up. If you see someone wriggling around on the bench as they try to press with their legs flapping around, they are losing power. The more stability you can create when you press, the stronger you will be."

What should I do if I am struggling with performing the bench press well?

You should perform the bench press more than once to help you gain more practice during the movement. You can perfect the technique by using lighter loads, for instance using roughly 70-80% of your 1RM.

Deadlift

From the toe to your head, many muscles are involved. Deadlifting if done properly can strengthen every area from the traps to your calves. Nevertheless, doing it wrong, can mess you up badly. Because many muscles are involved, it is a perfect way of losing fat while building the muscle mass because of the high demands placed on the body.

How do you rate?

- Beginner 1.5 x Bodyweight

- Intermediate 2 x Bodyweight

- Advanced 2.5 x Bodyweight

What is the Perfect form?

Beginning with your feet shoulder-width apart, hold the bar using an overhand grip. Position the bar in such a way that your shoulders are over it while directly above your middle foot. To start the movement, ensure you pull your shoulders backward to activate your lats. During this process ensure your hamstrings are loaded while you pull the bar above the ground by straightening your legs. Once the bar goes above your knees, you should straighten up pending when you are standing upright after which you reverse your movement backward. Since you are starting as a beginner if you consider it very heavy, you may drop the bar but it has to be careful.

Expert tip

According to an expert in powerlifting, "Keep the barbell close," because "Holding a heavyweight close to the body makes it much easier to lift. And your starting position should be with the bar covering the knot in your shoelaces."

How people get it wrong?

During lifting, they do it using a rounded back. Three reasons necessities this mistake – they lack the mobility to lift from the floor through a good back position, bad technique or too much weight on the bar.

What should I do if I am struggling with performing the deadlift well?

For those who are having difficulty in maintaining a good back position during the pulling process from the floor, they should consider elevating the barbell in the rack. This will help in reducing the mobility requirement while helping to maintain the accurate position. As you continue to practice, try as much as possible to minimize the height of the lift you pull.

POWERLIFTING ROUTINE FOR BEGINNERS AND EXPERIENCE LIFTERS

As a beginner in powerlifting setting up a powerlifting routine is very important if you really take your training seriously. This routine if properly set up will be one of the most demanding and intense forms of weightlifting. However, it comprises of little exercises, which is completed with some effort. By now, you are aware that powerlifting comprises of three lifts that are normally performed in the gym. These are the deadlifts, the squats, and the bench presses. Nevertheless, there are certain things to keep in mind regarding your powerlifting training.

Exercise Selection

The choice of exercise for your powerlifting routine is comparatively direct. Resistance exercises can be grouped either as core or assistance exercise. Core exercise involves the recruiting of one or more large muscles groups like the shoulders, chest or quadriceps. The assistance exercises involve the recruiting of the smaller muscle groups like the calf muscles, trapezius, and the biceps.

Though you can incorporate these two exercises into your powerlifting workout, the prominence must be on the core exercises with the deadlifts, bench presses and squats taking higher priority.

Training Frequency

It is important to note that the number of sessions per week will differ from 2 to a maximum of 6 depending on the structure of the powerlifting routine. Competitive powerlifting comprises of the lifting of maximum loads. There is a split routine adopted by most powerlifting programs, which give room for the different muscle groups to be worked in different days.

Training Load & Repetitions

Powerlifting isn't the same as bodybuilding, it involves maximal effort for a single rep and your training should demonstrate this. You may think that the ability to produce maximum strength depends largely on the cross-sectional area of the muscle size but this is just half of the truth. It also depends on your ability to recruit and synchronize every twitch fiber needed in the action.

Volume

This is the total amount of weight lifted during a series of training sessions. There are signs that singles sets increase the maximal strength of untrained individuals. Nevertheless, for experienced lifters, there is need to use higher volumes to promote further strength gains. According to studies, if you perform 3 sets without any failure in each set, this enhances strength to a greater degree when compared to a set performed to failure.

SAMPLE POWERLIFTING PROGRAM

In this section is a sample-powerlifting program for a single phase (6-10 weeks) of training through a long-term powerlifting routine. You must complete an anatomical adaptation routine as a beginner for a minimum of 8 weeks prior to you moving to this program. Such routine would incorporate more exercises to prep every ligament, joints, and connective tissue for more intense training.

Note: This program doesn't put into consideration the variation in training load and volume that experienced lifters will benefit from.

Sample Powerlifting Routine

DAY 1	Set 1	Set 2	Set 3	Set 4	Rest Interval
Squats (core)	90% × 3	90% × 3	90% × 3	100% × 3	3-5min

Dead Lifts (core)   80% × 4   80% × 4   85% × 3   90% × 2   3-5min

Leg Curls or Lunges (assistance)   70% × 3   70% × 10   70% × 10   70% ×
10   3-5min

Weighted Crunches (assistance)   10-12   10-12   10-12   10-12   3-5min

DAY 2

Bench Presses(core)   90% × 3   90% × 3   95% × 2   100% × 1   3-5min

Bent Over Rows (assistance) 70% × 10   70% × 10   70% × 10   70% × 10
        3-5min

Shoulder Presses(core)   90% × 3   90% × 3   95% × 2   95% × 2
        3-5min

Triceps Extension(assistance) 70% × 10   70% × 10   70% × 10   70% × 10
        3-5min

The routine in the image above would be completed in 4 sessions per week. For instance, Monday = Day 1, Tuesday = Day 2, Wednesday = Rest Day, Thursday = Repeat Day 1, Friday = Repeat Day 2, Saturday & Sunday = Rest Days.

Note: There are no warm-up sets included in the sets above. You should complete two or three sets of at least 8-10 reps before each exercise.

Sample for a 30-Day Beginner Challenge

Day 1

Pushups: 5

Squats:50

Sit-ups: 10

Lunges: 20

Day 2

Pushups: 5

Squats:55

Sit-ups: 15

Lunges: 21

Day 3

Pushups: 7

Squats:60

Sit-ups: 15

Lunges: 22

Day 4

Pushups: 7

Squats: Rest

Sit-ups: 25

Lunges: 23

Day 5

Pushups: 8

Squats:70

Sit-ups: 30

Lunges: Rest

Day 6

Pushups: 9

Squats:75

Sit-ups: 35

Lunges: 25

Day 7

Pushups: Rest

Squats:80

Sit-ups: Rest

Lunges: 26

Day 8

Pushups: 8

Squats: Rest

Sit-ups: 45

Lunges: 27

Day 9

Pushups: 9

Squats:100

Sit-ups: 45

Lunges: 28

Day 10

Pushups:10

Squats:105

Sit-ups: 50

Lunges: 29

Day 11

Pushups:10

Squats:110

Sit-ups: 55

Lunges: Rest

Day 12

Pushups:12

Squats: Rest

Sit-ups: 55

Lunges: 31

Day 13

Pushups:12

Squats:130

Sit-ups: Rest

Lunges: 32

Day 14

Pushups: Rest

Squats:135

Sit-ups: 60

Lunges: 33

Day 15

Pushups:13

Squats:140

Sit-ups: 65

Lunges: 34

Day 16

Pushups:15

Squats: Rest

Sit-ups:65

Lunges:35

Day 17

Pushups:16

Squats:150

Sit-ups: 70

Lunges: 36

Day 18

Pushups:16

Squats:155

Sit-ups: 70

Lunges: Rest

Day 19

Pushups:19

Squats:160

Sit-ups: 75

Lunges: 38

Day 20

Pushups:21

Squats: Rest

Sit-ups: 75

Lunges: 38

Day 21

Pushups: Rest

Squats:180

Sit-ups:75

Lunges: 40

Day 22

Pushups:23

Squats:185

Sit-ups: Rest

Lunges:41   Day 23

Pushups:26

Squats:190

Sit-ups: 80

Lunges: 42   Day 24

Pushups:28

Squats: Rest

Sit-ups: 80

Lunges: 43   Day 25

Pushups:30

Squats:220

Sit-ups:85

Lunges: Rest   Day 26

Pushups:32

Squats:225

Sit-ups: 85

Lunges: 45   Day 27

Pushups:34

Squats:230

Sit-ups: 90

Lunges: 46   Day 28

Pushups:37

Squats: Rest

Sit-ups: Rest

Lunges: 46

Day 29

Pushups:38

Squats:240

Sit-ups:95 Lunges:45

Day 30

Pushups:40

Squats:250

Sit-ups:100

Lunges: 50

COMMON BEGINNERS POWERLIFTING MISTAKES AND HOW TO AVOID THEM

You cannot reverse a mistake once you make it. However, you can learn from some. As a beginner in powerlifting training, it is hard for you not to make mistakes. We all make mistakes but the painful aspect is not learning from the mistake. Instead, we repeat them. As a beginner in powerlifting, you are bound to make mistakes in your quest of becoming stronger and bigger.

The following are some of the mistakes to be corrected if many advanced powerlifters knew have someone informed them. Instead of making the mistakes, you have the tips to avoid such mistakes. Without further ado, let us begin!

Master the lifting techniques

One cannot overstress this enough. The technique is very important when it comes to powerlifting. The wrong technique will create injuries, which is why you must do everything possible to practice or work on every technique.

Don't work out more than twice a week

The principle is that less work out is great. Working twice per week is a good start and it gives you more time to rest and get things done when you ought to.

No explosive lifting

If your goal as a beginner is to do powerlifting as a lifetime thing, having a healthy body without injury is not an option. You need to perform reps deliberately and on a constant rate.

Consume 5-6 small meals daily

This meal should include potato chips, greasy burgers, and frozen pizza. Eating a balanced diet is very important while doing your fitness routine. In the next chapter, we will explore the importance of diet to your fitness goal. Don't make the mistake of going to the gym without stepping up your diet. You need the right amount of "fuel" to power your muscle. In line with this, ensure you spend your money on quality food rather than fad supplements

Avoid these exercises

Don't make the mistake of performing the following exercises – cambered bar bench press, bench press to the neck, press behind neck, and stiffed-legged deadlifts.

Don't train like it is for a competition

This mistake is committed by most beginners who began their training with the mindset of doing it for a competition. Many trainees train like competitive lifters who use heavy weights and low reps frequently. Doing this will take a toll on your body and you may not see the overall effect on your body now.

Perform one work set for each exercise

What is the stress if the job can be done in a set?

Perform no more than 6-7 exercises in a single time

Your goal as a beginner is to concentrate your effort on the basic exercises. Master each technique used in performing these exercises. Even if you are using a program, it shouldn't be so complicated for it to be effective. Most times, the simplest programs are the most productive.

Put a check to your ego

Your ego as a beginner is your worst enemy. The macho bull showed by most experts if followed will likely get you into serious trouble. Don't allow your ego be a guiding force to your lifting.

Keep a comprehensive training log

This is very important because you will need something to show your progress. The biggest mistake you will make as a beginner is not having or keeping a comprehensive log of your training. Do you remember your first weight? Did you remember the weight you did 13 weeks ago? How do you measure your progress if these questions cannot be answered? Start today by keeping a detailed training log.

Don't focus your training on short-term but long-term

Don't try to get as much muscle gains in a short time. Trying to progress as fast as possible give room for injuries. Avoid the temptation of adding weight very quickly. Always be patient during your training.

Use fractional weight plates

This point is directly related to the previous point talked about. Long-term should be the focus. For instance, how can you expect to increase 4 pounds per week in the squat for a year? Imagine 4 pounds per week for 52 weeks will give 208 pounds. Assuming you are squatting 240 by 20 today, is it possible to squat 500 by 20 in a year? Let us face it this is not possible. Dust your ego and use small plates. You can start with a pound or less. Little by little, you can then increase it.

Don't arch during the bench press.

If you arch during your bench press, you are not building your muscle but merely demonstrating strength. Apart from this, it is also dangerous to the lower back of your body.

Get enough sleep

Sleep is a very important aspect of your recovery process. Don't take watching the late show to be of more priority over the health benefits of you having a good night rest. If you don't get enough sleep, you will surely short-circuit your efforts in the gym.

Don't purchase a muscle comic book.

Most beginners are a victim of this. They fantasize about people with great physiques and this makes them to buy comic books. A note of warning, these muscle comic books only provide unrealistic expectations. Most of the physiques attained by these bodybuilders in the comic books or magazines are obtainable by few individuals.

CHAPTER FOUR: NUTRITION AND FITNESS

Irrespective of the amount of effort you put into your training, without the right nutrition, you are just wasting your time. No matter how hard you try or invest so much time in the gym without the proper nutrition, you are simply holding back your progress. Do you still need some sort of convincing on the importance of nutrition to fitness? Well, in this section, you will learn some important keys to unlocking your training through nutrition. No training explained from the beginning of this eBook will profit you without a good nutrition guide. So, what is the importance of nutrition in fitness?

Health and Wellbeing

Your primary focus must be on optimizing your health before considering any performance goal like building your muscle. A healthy athlete has the chance of performing well. When you eat for health, it means your diet will contain different varieties of vegetables and fruits. It will include healthy fats, dairy products, and whole grains. You can avoid chronic health conditions such as type 2 diabetes, cholesterol, heart disease, and obesity when you avoid foods with high fat, sugar, and salt.

Improve strength training

Nutrition helps in recovery and strength training. Consuming protein-rich meals during your training period will help provide recovery for your tired muscles. With this, you get back to the gym refreshed and energized to continue your training. Muscle recovery needs different minerals and vitamins that come from the nutritious foods we consume. When you have a well-structured meal plan – like the one implemented in this eBook- and integrated into your training routine, this will improve your training performance.

Your Nutrition Plan

If you are going to stay healthy or lose fat, there is need to have a special meal plan to actualize your fitness goal. To help you, we have created a 30 days meal plan to reach your fitness goal. You have no option but to stock, your pantry and fridge with foods outline in the grocery lists of this eBook. Remember the composition of each of this meal will largely depend on what your fitness goal is.

Grocery List

For starters, you will need more of starchy carbs and fewer fats after and before each workout to promote muscle growth and energy. For those training just to get more pack on size, you will have to eat more frequently.

You will need to eat more starchy carbs and fewer fats before and after workouts to promote energy and muscle growth. If you are training to pack on size, you'll eat like this more frequently. And when your hours removed from a workout, you'll limit starches and increase fats, which will keep you on track to meet your fat-loss goals. For meals containing starchy carbohydrates, your meal options include:

Meals Containing Starchy Carbohydrates

Starch Wraps, cereals, bread, whole-wheat pasta, oats, potatoes, yam, quinoa, and brown rice

Protein Greek yogurt, white fish, white meat, whole eggs (sparingly), egg whites, and protein powders

Fruits/Vegetables/Legumes   Beans, Green or fibrous vegetables, and Tropical Fruits

Oil   Use sparingly not tablespoons but teaspoons.

Meals Not Containing Starchy Carbohydrates

Protein Greek Yogurt, white fish or oily fish, red meat, white meat, eggs, and protein Powders

Fruits/vegetables/legumes   Beans, green/fibrous, berries

Oil   Full-fat cheeses, canola mayonnaise, coconut oil, nuts/seeds, and Avocadoes

PILLARS OF NUTRITION

Limit Processed Foods: Even if it comes in a bag, a carton or a box, if it has a brand name or label, it is likely processed and not worth consuming. Remove nutrient poor and high-calorie food from your diet plan.

Eat Six times a day: This is vital for beginners because you need to fuel your body with snacks and multiple small meals daily. This will help in keeping your blood-sugar level under control, stimulating the production of new muscle while stabilizing your metabolism.

Stay Hydrated: Consume as much water not forgetting that you need calorie-free beverages to keep your performance at its peak in the gym. Avoid sugar-laden drinks because it will sabotage your body's antioxidant defense and fatten your waistline.

Strategic Carbs: Carbs comes in two forms:

- Starchy – these include pasta, bread, and rice, which raise blood sugar quickly.

- Non-starchy carbs – These include whole grains, vegetables, and fruits, which have a high content of fiber but raise the blood sugar gradually.

The non-starchy carbs hardly a problem so enjoy them. Nevertheless, the timing of when you eat starchy carbs is crucial, as it is the key to getting a muscular and lean body. The best time to eat them is directly after workouts or in the morning.

Lean Protein: The best sources of lean protein include soy, lower-fat dairy foods, fish, chicken, and lean beef. In as much as whole foods should be your primary option, you can use a good protein powder with your diet to get the required protein macros needed for the day. You may also consider adding whey protein while using a slow digesting casein protein to speed up your weight.

NUTRITION AND STRENGTH TRAINING

Perhaps you have devoted so much time to the gym trying as much as possible to build your muscle through strength training, however, the outcome may not be pleasant if you neglect the place of proper diet.

Integrating a proper diet plan into your strength training will enable you to actualize your goal by providing maximum nutrition and calories. Eating properly can help you derive a sculpted and lean body. Then what is the role of protein in all these.

Role of Protein in Strength Training

A diet, which supports an active strength training routine, must contain more protein than your standard diet. The suggested daily protein allowed is 0.8g per kilogram of the body weight for an average person. Nevertheless, for a person who is actively involved in strength training and with the intent of building their muscle should take between 1.4 to 2.4g of protein per kilogram of the body weight. This is the recommended daily consumption needed.

Other Macronutrients

In as much as there is high emphasizes on a high protein diet for people undergoing strength training, fats and carbohydrates are still important. Carbohydrate is needed to provide energy for your daily activity and workouts. For those weighing more than 200 lbs. your minimum consumption should be between 40 to 55 g for each meal. For those whose weight is between 150 to 190 lbs., 30 to 35 g per meal is perfect.

Types of Foods

Lean proteins such as lean beef, egg whites, whey protein, fish, and white-meat poultry have low saturated fat and provide a complete amino acid for the body. Healthy carbohydrates such as fruits, vegetables, and whole grains provide the best fiber and nutrition for the body. Unsaturated fats do not create health problem as Trans fats and saturated fats do. However, they provide support for strength training by helping with hormone production and vitamin absorption.

What is the strategy for diet regarding strength training?

Instead of overloading nutrition and calories at the three meals, your strength training diet should comprise of multiple smaller meals, which is consumed every three to four hours daily. This is necessary, as it will help in maximizing your nutrient intake while keeping you from becoming too hungry.

Every meal must contain a healthy carbohydrate and protein. Examples of meals are broccoli and olive oil, grilled chicken with brown rice or flax seed with milk. Ensure each of these meals are split and consumed before and after each strength training workout. This will help in muscle repair and growth.

30 DAYS MEAL PLAN

A sample meal plan for five consecutive days, which can be repeated for the next thirty days.

	Monday	Tuesday	Wednesday	Thursday	Friday

Meal 1

- ½-cup oatmeal (dry amount) prepared with water

- ½-cup strawberries

- 6 egg whites, cooked with 1 yolk

- 6 egg whites cooked with 1 yolk

- 1 medium bagel with 2 tbsp. reduced-fat peanut butter   •   ½-cup oatmeal prepared with water.

- 6 egg whites cooked with 1 yolk.

- 1 piece fruit   •   1 cup 1% milk

- 1 piece fruit

- 1 cup whole-grain cereal

- 1 Tbsp. peanut butter • 7 egg whites cooked with 1 yolk

- ½ cup strawberries

- ½ cup oatmeal made with water

Meal 2 • 1 Cup green vegetables

- 8 oz. chicken breast • 6 oz. chicken breast

- 1 cup green veggies

- 1 cup brown long-grain rice • 8 oz. chicken breast

- 1 cup green veggies • 1 cup green veggies

- Large baked potato with skin (3-4 inches in diameter)

- 6 oz. chicken breast • 8 oz. chicken breast

- 1 cup green veggies

Meal 3 Tuna sandwich prepared with 6-oz. can tuna (in spring water), 2 leaves romaine lettuce, 1 Tbsp. fat-free mayo, 2 slices whole-wheat bread • 6 oz. lean steak

- 1 cup green veggies • 6 oz. lean steak

- 1 cup green veggies

- Large baked potato with skin (3-4inches in diameter) • 6 oz. lean steak

- 1 cup green veggies

- Large baked potato with skin (3-4 inches in diameter) • 8 oz. sliced turkey

- 1 cup green veggies

- Large baked potato with skin (3-4 inches in diameter)

Meal 4 Protein shake prepared with 40g whey protein • Protein shake prepared with 30-40g whey protein • Low-carb, low-sugar protein bar • Protein shake made with 30-40 g whey protein • Protein shake prepared with 30-40g whey protein and 1 cup berries

Meal 5 Chicken salad made with 8 oz. chicken breast, ½ medium tomato, 2 Tbsp. Italian dressing, ½ cup broccoli, 2 leaves romaine lettuce   •   1 cup broccoli

•   8 oz. red snapper or halibut   •   Omelet made with 8 egg whites and 1 yolk, cooked with ½ cup broccoli, 2 mushrooms, fresh salsa   •   6-8 stalks asparagus

•   16-oz. can tuna (in spring water) made with 1 Tbsp fat-free mayo

•   6-8 stalks asparagus

•   7 oz. lean steak

Nutrient Estimate   1,817 calories, 255 g protein, 98 g carbohydrate, 37 g fat, and 20 g fiber   1,959, 254 g protein, 132 g carbohydrate, 39 g fat, and 17 g fiber   1,862 calories, 226 g protein, 149 g carbohydrate, 35 g fat, and 23 g fiber   1,984 calories, 226 g protein, 200 g carbohydrate, 29 g fat, 28 g fiber.   1,846 calories, 358 g protein, 122 g carbohydrate, 32 g fat, and 23 g fiber

CONCLUSION

Today, more people are becoming conscious of health and fitness. Nothing is as important as fitness and health for any human being. Not forgetting the fact that an unhealthy person will not enjoy life to its fullness. In this eBook, we have guided you on a key important aspect of keeping fit through powerlifting, bodybuilding and strength training.

Towards the ending, the importance of nutrition and fitness was highlighted. We need to eat fresh and green vegetables, eggs, fresh fruits, milk, etc. Our body requires sufficient amount of vitamin, mineral, and protein to be healthy and fit on a daily basis. The important aspect of this eBook is incorporating everything you have learned into your fitness and diet plan. Surely, you will be among those with the perfect body.

-- Mortuza Karzon